How To Improve Mental Patterns Happy Mindset

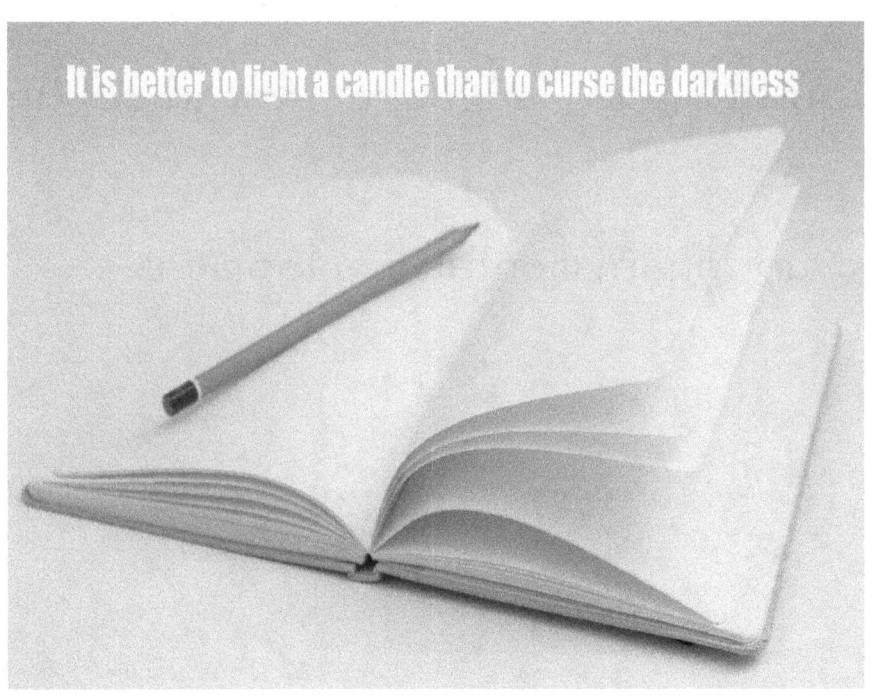

Jean Piaget

The period between birth and the

acquisition of language is marked by

extraordinary mental development.

As soon as he comes into this world,

the newborn baby opens his eyes to

observe everything that is happening

around him, but in reality he has no

perception of the world. We

understand that this outside world is

something that remains foreign to him

Because, we don't know how he

integrates it into his representations.

All that we know it is that it unites its

first bonds with its mother in a word Its

first contact with the world is done in a

family medium more precisely using its

mother. We believe that this phase is of

great importance in the mental

organization of the newborn."Each

child is endowed with characters

(characters) which are specific to him

and which must be taken into account if

we want his education to succeed: To

transmit a simple message to him, his

mother uses a limited number of words

accompanied by a few gestures, in

Indeed, each word will be listed in a

folder and the folder itself will be

inserted into a file, the processing of

words is done gradually inside its own

brain. Let us know here that the

external elements and the environment

play an important role and exert an

influence on the brain. Moreover, we

believe that the best way to address

one's children is based on reason and

logic, remember here that modern man

has deployed all his potential to

encourage his fellow human beings to

recognize certain decisions as true or

necessary, yet he adopted several ways

to rely on tangible arguments. Modern

man has grasped the primordial role of

ideas in the realization of his exploits.

Thus, it is essential to affirm that this

world is going to know a great

revolution because the one who

maintains the language has the power.

and the one who has no experience, has

nothing. In this perspective, we believe

that this kind of person will have the

ability to influence in his environment,

he will also be able to defend his own

interests Communication was never a

simple game between a transmitter and

a receiver, on the contrary it offers a

space decisive in establishing links

between the objectives to be achieved

and the results to be achieved. In

addition, man tended to use the

different aspects of language to

highlight his emotions, his fears and

ambitions. However, it should be noted

that argumentation, as a job that seems

very complicated, has today taken on a

large dimension in interactions with

others because it has dominated his

personal and collective universe. Later,

his gaze will focus on the purposes

knowing that language forms two major

entities: the first is that of the sender as

he has designed it and the second is

that of the receiver, as he wants to

embody it. , in other words the man

understands that he is solely

responsible for his own actions. These

are jointly related to his thoughts.

Therefore, we believe that it is

necessary to examine the power of

thoughts to understand its impact on

social life, likewise, it seems essential to

take a look at the world of thought

because in most cases it is better to

choose your words as you choose your

own clothes. But the problem that we

face today 'that is to say in the

mediatization of speeches and that

ideas are like the wind they do not have

a worship or a form, they are invisible

but one can feel their impact on the

individual and his entourage

We should also know that human

beings are always in a hurry, they don't

take all the time they need to check

their thoughts; attraction, seduction

open small doors for ideas regardless

of the content or the corpus or the

message

The child lives within his small family.

He hardly ceases to imitate those close

to him, especially his parents. The

acquisition of the gestures of the words

is done in the first years. According to

John Locke the newborn looks like a

blank sheet. you can write anything in

this sheet. all our ideas come

fromexperience, that is to say the set of

"observations that we make on external

and sensible objects, or on the interior

operations of our soul, which we

perceive and on which we reflect

ourselves" and which "provide our mind

the materials of all its thoughts. We are

the first responsible for our children.

Some parents wonder why their child

acts in an incomprehensible way

Every day we meet several people, our

discussion is based on multiple themes

or several subjects these try many times

to integrate their emotions, their

problems in the different conversations

sometimes only one idea could catch

your attention suppose that a young

man thirty-year-old tries to tell you

about his own experience with the sale

of several hundredof EBOOK. The

first question that traces its way into

consciousness would be how did it

achieve this goal? .In my opinion, this

experience would have a positive impact

on your future. The first idea that

comes to mind. I would like to become

like him a simple discussion with this man

awakens in you a certain positive

energy: ambition, will, success. Unlike if

you meet another person who talks to

you about betrayal. You read in his

eyes the sadness, the tendency to take

revenge, the contempt and the anger. In

short, the world of ideas is like a mirror

that helps you see everything that is

happening in your universe or it takes

you into the world of darkness. Know

that some ideas are like poison. they

need quick action or they poison your

mind and body, making it difficult for

people to recover from the shock.

Moreover, the complexity of ideas

resides in their multidimensional aspect

which affects the unconscious.

Because some ideas are stuck in the

habitus they guide us in our choices as

well as in our daily life, that is why we

must be vigilant when issuing certain

ideas. Never let negative ideas

dominate your daily life. Avoid listening

and seeing what is not right. For his

part, Paul Thiry d'Holbach emphasizes

the importance of the influence of the

social environment on the thought of

the human brain as being only "soft wax,

capable of receiving all the impressions

that one wants to make there. the

complexity of ideas resides in their

multidimensional aspect which affects

the unconscious. Because some ideas

are stuck in the habitus they guide us in

our choices as well as in our daily life,

that is why we must be vigilant when

issuing certain ideas. Never let negative

ideas dominate your daily life. Avoid

listening and seeing what is not right.

For his part, Paul Thiry d'Holbach

emphasizes the importance of the

influence of the social environment on

the thought of the human brain as being

only "soft wax, capable of receiving all

the impressions that one wants to make

there. the complexity of ideas resides in

their multidimensional aspect which

affects the unconscious. Because

some ideas are stuck in the habitus they

guide us in our choices as well as in our

daily life, that is why we must be vigilant

when issuing certain ideas. Never let

negative ideas dominate your daily life.

Avoid listening and seeing what is not right. For his part, Paul Thiry d'Holbach emphasizes the importance of the influence of the social environment on the thought of the human brain as being only "soft wax, capable of receiving all the impressions that one wants to make there. Because

some ideas are stuck in the habitus they

guide us in our choices as well as in our

daily life, that is why we must be vigilant

when issuing certain ideas. Never let

negative ideas dominate your daily life.

Avoid listening and seeing what is not

right. For his part, Paul Thiry

d'Holbach emphasizes the importance

of the influence of the social

environment on the thought of the

human brain as being only "soft wax,

capable of receiving all the impressions

that one wants to make there. Because

some ideas are stuck in the habitus they

guide us in our choices as well as in our

daily life, that is why we must be vigilant

when issuing certain ideas. Never let

negative ideas dominate your daily life.

Avoid listening and seeing what is not

right. For his part, Paul Thiry

d'Holbach emphasizes the importance

of the influence of the social

environment on the thought of the

human brain as being only "soft wax,

capable of receiving all the impressions

that one wants to make there.

Most people are not aware of the

gravity of the world of ideas, they

recognize their importance in

communication by saying that they

fillmultiple functions,But the reality is

that some ideas can ruin a society. We

also think that the idea as an entity has

an abstract nature. This nature refers

more precisely to two types of

knowledge: empirical knowledge and

scientific knowledge. In other words,

the world of ideas resembles a large

ocean that attracts many visitors. The

first do not know that this ocean is

deep and many people have succumbed

the second are a little attentive

Attachment: Small children are deeply

attached to their parents. They watch

their behavior carefully. Parents must

be attentive to this attachment, they

must explain to their children that the

family is a united group of belonging,

composed of those who will have to

help me without thinking

Trust: Trust is an essential quality, it is

built from the bonds that unite people.

Parents are called upon to help their

children build this quality, and to do so

they are invited to put their children in

learning situations to check whether

their children have acquired this skill.

Encouragement: To meet the challenges and achieve great feats, parents are invited to encourage their children, a successful effort should never go unnoticed on the contrary. He must be rewarded: Buy a gift, celebrate this event. Children need his gestures to feel the sense of success. Otherwise

their efforts are worth nothing.

Jean Piaget

Quote

1 - Intelligence is not what you know but what

you do when you don't know.

<u>Jean Piaget</u>

<u>Quote</u>

2- To invent is to combine mental schemes,

i.e. representative.

www.ingramcontent.com/pod-product-compliance
Lightning Source LLC
Chambersburg PA
CBHW072236230526
45466CB00024B/2082